UNDERSTANDING

IRON

AND BENEFITS

A Guide To Understanding Its Role In Health And Wellness, Key Targets, Focus Areas, And Transformative Advantages For Body And Mind

DR. LACEY MICHELLE

Disclaimer:

The information provided in this book is for general informational purposes only and is not intended as medical advice.

Readers are encouraged to consult with a qualified healthcare professional for any health concerns or questions.

The author of this book is not affiliated with any individual, website, organization, or products mentioned within.

This book does not endorse or promote any specific brands, services, or external entities. Any references made are purely for illustrative purposes and should not be construed as endorsements.

Readers are responsible for their own decisions and should conduct their own research before making any health-related choices.

Any liability resulting from the use of this information, whether direct or indirect, is disclaimed by the author and publisher.

Contents

About The Book

To sum up

Take a tour through the complex realm of iron supplementation and learn about the essential function it plays in preserving health and well-being. With the help of this book, you should be able to make well-informed decisions and get the knowledge necessary to move toward optimal health.

CHAPTER ONE

Iron Supplement Types

Iron deficiency anemia is frequently treated with iron supplements, which also help the body maintain normal iron levels. There are numerous varieties of iron supplements available, and each has unique properties and rates of absorption. Comprehending the distinctions among these kinds is essential for efficient supplementing.

Non-Heme Vs. Heme Iron

The two main types of dietary iron are heme iron and non-heme iron, which vary in their sources and rates of absorption.

Foods derived from animals, such as red meat, chicken, and fish, contain heme iron. It comes from the proteins found in muscle and blood called myoglobin and hemoglobin. Heme iron is frequently regarded as the most bioavailable type of iron due to its high absorption rate by the body.

Conversely, plant-based diets and fortified goods include non-heme iron. Compared to heme iron, this form of iron is less readily absorbed.

Several factors, including dietary components like phytates and tannins that can hinder the uptake of non-heme iron, can affect how well it is absorbed.

It is frequently advised to take non-heme iron with foods high in vitamin C since this can aid in the conversion of ferric iron (Fe^{3+}) into ferrous iron (Fe^{2+}), a form that is easier to absorb.

Iron: Ferrous versus Ferric

Ferrous iron and ferric iron are the two primary chemical types of iron that are accessible as supplements. Iron is found in the Fe^{2+} state in ferrous iron supplements and the Fe^{3+} state in ferric iron supplements. Their bioavailability and the degree to which the body absorbs them are the main distinctions between the two.

In comparison to ferric iron, ferrous iron is typically thought to be more bioavailable and easier for the body to absorb.

This is why ferrous iron compounds like ferrous fumarate, gluconate, and sulfate are used in the formulation of many iron supplements.

Since these substances are more successful in treating iron deficiency anemia, they are frequently utilized.

Even though they are less absorbable, ferric iron supplements might still be useful for augmenting iron levels.

They are frequently utilized in cases where people have gastrointestinal problems or adverse reactions to ferrous iron supplements. Healthcare providers may also recommend slow-release or extended-release ferric iron supplements to lower adverse effects and increase tolerability.

Various Iron Supplement Forms

There are numerous types of iron supplements available, each with special qualities and benefits. Ferrous fumarate, ferrous gluconate, ferrous sulfate, and ferric poly maltose are a few typical types.

One of the most popular iron supplements is ferrous sulfate, which comes in tablet and liquid form. To reduce stomach discomfort, taking it with food is frequently advised.

Another popular form of iron supplement is ferrous gluconate, which is thought to have less severe adverse effects than ferrous sulfate.

You can take it with or without meals. Although ferrous fumarate is a more concentrated type of iron that enables smaller pill sizes, some people may have more digestive pain from it.

Those with more severe iron deficiency anemia or those who cannot take oral iron supplements can receive ferric poly maltose, a ferric iron complex, intravenously. It is given under a doctor's supervision.

To meet the demands, tastes, and tolerance levels of each individual, iron supplements are available in a variety of formats. A person should select an iron supplement based on the existence of other minerals or dietary components that may affect iron absorption, as well as characteristics like side effects and absorption rates.

Speaking with a medical expert can assist in figuring out the best kind and amount of iron supplement for a person's unique situation.

Iron Shortfall:

A frequent nutritional condition known as iron insufficiency arises when the body does not get enough of this crucial element, which is necessary for many physiological processes. Hemoglobin, a protein in red blood cells that carries oxygen from the lungs to the rest of the body, is formed primarily by iron.

Iron deficiency anemia is a disorder that can result from the body not having enough iron.

Knowing What Iron Deficiency Anemia Is

One particular kind of anemia called iron deficiency anemia is typified by a drop in red blood cell count and oxygen-carrying capacity.

When there is not enough iron available to make enough hemoglobin, this disease develops. The body finds it difficult to transfer oxygen when there is insufficient functional hemoglobin, which can result in several health issues.

Reasons And Danger Factors:

Effective prevention and therapy of iron insufficiency require an understanding of the various factors that can contribute to the condition.

Dietary variables are important; one typical cause is a diet low in iron-rich foods, such as poultry, fish, red meat, and fortified cereals. Iron deficiency can also result from some medical diseases that affect the digestive system's ability to absorb iron, such as gastrointestinal operations, inflammatory bowel disease, and celiac disease. Due to increased iron demands, women—especially those who are pregnant or have heavy periods—are more likely to develop iron insufficiency.

Blood loss from wounds, operations, or long-term bleeding problems are additional risk factors. Because they might not consume as much heme iron (found in animal products) in their diets, vegetarians,ans and vegans should be especially careful to collect non-heme iron (found in plant-based sources) and, if needed, think about supplementing.

Signs And Prognosis:

While iron deficiency anemia can present with a variety of symptoms, it is important to identify the condition early on because these symptoms frequently worsen over time. Weakness, exhaustion, pale complexion, breathing difficulties, cold hands and feet, brittle nails, and an elevated risk of infection are typical symptoms.

These symptoms are brought on by low hemoglobin levels, which reduce the blood's ability to deliver oxygen.

Healthcare professionals usually do blood tests to diagnose iron deficiency anemia. These tests may measure serum iron levels, ferritin levels, and transferrin saturation.

To measure hemoglobin, hematocrit, and red blood cell count, a complete blood count (CBC) is also frequently carried out.

These tests assist medical practitioners in confirming the diagnosis and assessing the severity of the ailment.

Iron supplementation and dietary changes are frequently used to treat iron deficiency anemia once it has been identified.

The precise course of treatment may change based on the underlying causes and unique medical circumstances.

If a more serious underlying issue is the cause of the iron shortage, treating the underlying cause is essential to long-term health.

It's crucial to follow up with a healthcare professional regularly to assess progress and make any therapy adjustments.

When prescribed, iron supplements are often taken carefully, taking into account the right amount and length of time to prevent toxicity or adverse effects.

Iron-Powder Foods

Iron is a vital mineral for human health, as it is involved in many physiological functions, chiefly the synthesis of hemoglobin, the red blood cell protein that carries oxygen throughout the body.

A lack of iron can cause anemia, weariness, weakness, and other health problems. Thus, it's critical to maintain an appropriate iron intake, and eating foods high in iron is one method to do this.

Bioavailability and Absorption of Iron

As a component of hemoglobin and myoglobin, iron is an important mineral that is vital for many physiological processes in the human body, most notably its role in oxygen delivery. However, several factors that affect iron's bioavailability might also affect the body's capacity to absorb and use it efficiently.

Affecting Factors for Iron Absorption

Source of Iron: Heme iron, which is found in animal products, and non-heme iron, which is found in plant-based sources, are the two kinds of iron that are found in food. Non-heme iron has a lower absorption rate of 2-20% whereas heme iron is more easily absorbed by the body, with an absorption rate of approximately 15-35%.

Iron Status: Depending on its present iron reserves, the body controls the absorption of iron. The body increases absorption when iron stores are low, but decreases absorption when iron stores are high or sufficient. The iron balance is preserved in part by this regulation.

Iron Supplements: The bioavailability of iron supplements varies depending on the kind, such as ferrous sulfate, ferrous gluconate, or other forms.

The iron absorption capacity of the body can be influenced by the kind and composition of the supplement.

Dietary Factors: Several dietary elements can affect how well iron is absorbed. Phytates, contained in whole grains and legumes, and polyphenols, prevalent in tea and coffee, can limit iron absorption. Conversely, vitamin C can improve the absorption of non-heme iron.

Digestive Health: Disorders that affect the digestive system, such as Crohn's disease, celiac disease, or surgery that modifies the digestive tract, might influence the absorption of iron. These factors might lessen the surface area available for absorption or interfere with the body's capacity to use the iron that has been absorbed.

Improving the Bioavailability of Iron

There are various methods to increase the bioavailability of non-heme iron from plant-based sources and iron supplements:

Iron and Vitamin C Together: Eating vitamin C-rich meals with non-heme iron sources can improve absorption. Non-heme iron is changed by vitamin C into a more soluble form that the body can absorb more easily.

Avoiding Inhibitors: It is best to take supplements or foods high in iron separately from foods high in phytates and polyphenols to reduce the interference these substances cause. Furthermore, grains and legumes can improve iron absorption and lower their phytate level by soaking, sprouting, or fermenting.

Cooking Techniques: The bioavailability of iron can be affected by specific cooking techniques. Soaking, boiling, or blanching vegetables, for instance, can lessen their concentration of compounds that prevent the absorption of iron.

Foods fortified with Iron: Adding iron to meals can be a useful strategy for raising iron consumption. To combat iron deficiency, fortifying staple foods like flour and cereals is a popular public health tactic.

Sufficient Consumption of Protein: Protein helps aid in the absorption of non-heme iron.

You can increase the bioavailability of iron in your diet by consuming foods high in protein.

Iron Poisoning And Its Repercussions

When the body accumulates too much iron, it can lead to iron toxicity, also known as iron overload. Numerous things, such as consuming too many meals high in iron, taking iron supplements for an extended period, or having underlying medical disorders that interfere with iron management, can cause this illness.

An excessive amount of iron in the body can have several negative effects.

The potential for iron overload to harm essential organs including the liver, heart, and pancreas is one of the main causes for concern.

Overconsumption of iron can produce dangerous free radicals that can damage cells and tissues by causing oxidative stress and inflammation. Depending on which organs are impacted, this damage may show up as diabetes, heart issues, or liver illness.

Iron overload can also affect the body's other systems. Endocrine disruption, skin pigmentation, and joint pain are possible outcomes.

The skin may turn gray or golden, which is a defining feature of hemochromatosis, a genetic illness linked to excessive absorption of iron. Hormonal abnormalities may result from issues with the endocrine system brought on by iron excess.

Tracking Hematitin Levels

Regularly checking iron levels is crucial, particularly for those who are taking iron supplements for medical conditions or are at risk of iron overload. Serum ferritin levels, which indicate the body's iron reserves, can be measured by blood tests for monitoring.

Further tests that can reveal important details regarding iron status include transferrin saturation and total iron-binding capacity.

These tests are used by doctors to evaluate patients' iron levels, establish if iron supplements are required, and spot any possible signs of iron overload. Optimizing health outcomes requires striking a balance between minimizing iron overload and deficiency.

Handling Too Much Iron

Two main strategies are usually used to manage iron overload: therapeutic phlebotomy and dietary adjustment. A medical treatment called therapeutic phlebotomy includes drawing a predetermined volume of blood to lower the body's iron levels. People with secondary hemochromatosis brought on by other medical disorders or those with hereditary hemochromatosis are frequently advised to adopt this technique.

Making dietary changes can also be very helpful in treating iron overload. People who have elevated iron levels might have to limit their use of foods high in iron, like red meat and cereals fortified with iron.

Furthermore, since vitamin C increases iron absorption, eliminating vitamin C supplements and foods high in nutrients can assist in lowering iron absorption.

In conclusion, while iron supplements are necessary for those with iron-deficiency anemia, it's critical to use them sparingly and by medical advice to avoid iron excess. The body's overabundance of iron can cause serious health problems, such as systemic illnesses and organ damage.

To prevent iron overload and achieve a balance between preventing deficiency, routine blood test monitoring of iron levels is crucial. Therapeutic phlebotomy and dietary modifications are commonly used to manage iron overload, providing efficient means of reducing excess iron in the body and minimizing related health hazards.

CHAPTER TWO

Natural Sources Of Iron For The Diet

There are two forms of dietary iron: heme iron and non-heme iron. Animal-based diets contain heme iron, which the body can absorb more readily.

Heme iron can be found, for instance, in fish, chicken, and red meat. Plant-based diets contain non-heme iron, which is less easily absorbed than heme iron. Good sources of non-heme iron include legumes, fortified cereals, nuts, seeds, and dark leafy greens.

Heme iron is primarily found in red meat, specifically in beef and The liver is one of the organ meats that has the highest iron content. Heme iron is also found in poultry and fish, such as salmon, turkey, and chicken, albeit in somewhat smaller amounts.

For those who follow a vegetarian or vegan diet, it's crucial to focus on non-heme iron sources including lentils, tofu, fortified cereals, beans, and spinach.

Increasing Uptake Of Iron

Plant-based foods should be consumed in conjunction with meals or substances that improve absorption to maximize the absorption of non-heme iron from them. For example, vitamin C can greatly enhance the absorption of non-heme iron.

Therefore, it's preferable to complement iron-rich plant foods with fruits like oranges, strawberries, or kiwi.

However, some drugs can prevent the body from absorbing iron.

These include tannins found in tea and coffee, as well as calcium and phytates present in some grains and legumes.

 It is advisable to stay away from taking these inhibitors with foods high in iron. Tea and coffee should be consumed separately from meals as they may decrease the absorption of iron.

Dietary Advice For Consuming Iron

Take into consideration implementing the following dietary advice into your daily routine to guarantee an adequate intake of dietary iron:

Balanced Diet: Make sure your diet is well-balanced and full of heme and non-heme foods that are high in iron.

This will satisfy your iron needs while assisting you in obtaining a greater variety of nutrients.

Cooking Methods: Take note of any techniques that may affect the amount of iron in food. Iron-rich foods that are overcooked or overboiled may lose some of their iron content, so use softer cooking methods like stir-frying or steaming instead.

Iron Supplements: People with certain medical disorders or iron deficiency may occasionally require iron supplements.

To ascertain the proper dosage and kind of iron supplements, speak with a healthcare provider before beginning any supplementation.

Consider the way that iron and other nutrients interact with one another. For example, foods high in calcium may hinder the absorption of iron; if you are concerned about your iron intake, avoid ingesting these items at the same time.

Dietary Restrictions: If you follow a vegetarian or vegan diet, plan your meals carefully to ensure appropriate iron consumption from plant-based sources. Be careful of potential absorption inhibitors and boosters.

Frequent Health Checkups: You can keep an eye on your general health and iron levels by scheduling regular health checkups. Seek advice and testing from a healthcare provider if you believe you may have an iron deficiency.

To sum up, keeping a sufficient intake of iron is essential for general health and well-being.

You can make sure your body gets the iron it needs to function at its best by including a variety of foods high in iron in your diet and being aware of circumstances that may improve or hinder iron absorption.

Iron deficiency can be avoided and general health can be enhanced by dietary decisions and educated habits.

CHAPTER THREE

Iron-Related Health Benefits:

The human body needs iron to function properly in several physiological activities. It is an essential part of hemoglobin, the red blood cell protein that carries oxygen from the lungs to the body's other tissues.

In addition, iron is involved in many enzymatic processes, DNA synthesis, and the generation of cellular energy.

Since both an excess and a shortage of iron can cause health issues, it is essential to maintain the proper balance of iron in the body for overall health. To treat deficiencies and avoid related health problems, iron supplements are frequently advised in situations when food consumption or absorption of iron is inadequate.

Who Requires Supplemental Iron?

Not everyone requires iron supplements, as the dietary intake of this mineral is normally adequate for most people. Many foods, such as red meat, chicken, fish, beans, lentils, fortified cereals, and dark leafy greens, naturally contain iron.

In actuality, getting enough iron from food is frequently simpler than getting it from supplements. Nonetheless, certain demographics may require iron supplements:

Iron-Deficiency Anemia: The most frequent cause of iron supplementation is this illness. Fatigue, weakness, and other symptoms are caused by lower-than-normal quantities of hemoglobin and red blood cells in people with iron-deficiency anemia.

To improve anemia and restore iron levels, doctors frequently prescribe iron supplements.

Pregnant Women: A woman's blood volume rises during pregnancy, and her body needs extra iron to support the developing placenta and fetus. To avoid iron-deficiency anemia during pregnancy, iron supplements are frequently advised.

Children: Iron supplements may be necessary to assist the growth and development of infants and early children who have inadequate iron intake or poor absorption.

Vegans and vegetarians: People who eat only plant-based meals may need to be particularly careful about how much iron they take in since the non-heme iron in these foods is not as easily absorbed as the heme iron found in animal products. For those who may be deficient, iron supplements may be of consideration.

People with Gastrointestinal Disorders: Iron absorption can be impacted by conditions such as Crohn's disease, gastric bypass surgery, and celiac disease. Supplements can be required in these situations to make up for the decreased absorption of iron.

Advantages And Dangers:

When used as directed, iron supplements have a host of positive health effects. They are very useful in treating iron-deficiency anemia, which promotes better cognitive function, more energy, and general well-being. Sustaining appropriate iron levels also helps to prevent infection and boost immunity.

However, since taking too much iron can be hazardous, it's imperative to consume supplements under a doctor's supervision. Hemochromatosis, or iron overload, can harm organs, especially the heart, liver, and pancreas. Iron supplement side effects that are frequently seen include nausea, constipation, and gastrointestinal distress. It's critical to adhere to suggested dosages and refrain from self-prescribing iron supplements to minimize the hazards connected with high iron levels.

Furthermore, some people—such as those with hemochromatosis or other genetic disorders affecting iron metabolism—may be more susceptible to negative effects from iron supplementation.

Therefore, speaking with a healthcare professional is essential to determining the right amount and determining whether iron supplementation is necessary.

Suggested Daily Amount:

The age, gender, and stage of life that determine the recommended daily allowance (RDA) for iron are all factors. The National Institutes of Health in the US determines the recommended daily allowance (RDA) for iron, which is as follows:

Infants aged 0 to 6 months: 0.27 mg

7–12 month-old infants: 11 mg

Children aged 1-3: 7 mg

Children aged 4 to 8: 10 mg

Children aged 9 to 13: 8 mg

For males aged 14 to 18: 11 mg

Girls aged 14 to 18: 15 mg

For males aged 19 and above: 8 mg

Women aged 19 to 50: 18 mg

For women aged 51 and beyond 8 mg

Ladies in pregnancy: 27 mg

Women who are nursing: 9–10 mg

It's crucial to remember that everyone has different demands when it comes to iron; depending on their unique situation, some people may need more or less iron. When someone has an iron deficiency, a medical practitioner will determine the right amount of supplements to suit their needs without putting them in danger of taking too much iron. To make sure that iron supplements are effectively treating deficiencies and promoting improved general health, regular monitoring and evaluation are required.

CHAPTER FOUR

Selecting The Appropriate Iron Supplement

Selecting the appropriate iron supplement requires research and careful consideration of several aspects. Iron deficiency anemia, which can arise from several factors including insufficient food intake, problems with malabsorption, or increased iron requirements because of pregnancy or excessive menstrual bleeding, is frequently treated or prevented using iron supplements. Choosing the best iron supplement requires knowledge of the kinds that are available, taking unique demographics into account, and determining whether over-the-counter and prescription solutions are best.

Iron Supplement Types

Iron supplements come in a variety of forms, and each has unique qualities. Ferrous fumarate, ferrous gluconate, ferrous sulfate, and ferric iron preparations are the most widely used types.

Because of its high elemental iron content, ferrous sulfate is the one that is most frequently given among these. It is significant to remember that the elemental iron concentration in each kind of supplement might differ, which can impact tolerability and absorption.

Ferrous sulfate, for example, has a larger proportion of elemental iron than ferrous gluconate.

Moreover, there are various forms of iron supplements available, including liquid, tablets, capsules, and intravenous choices.

Certain formulations may be preferred by some people due to their digestive health or the convenience of administration.

In severe circumstances, intravenous iron therapy may be advised for those who are unable to tolerate the gastrointestinal adverse effects of oral iron supplements.

Taking Special Populations Into Account
There may be particular demands and considerations for iron supplements for certain groups.

For example, pregnant women frequently need to consume more iron to support the growing fetus and increase blood volume. Thus, it may be advised to take specific iron supplements or prenatal vitamins containing iron while pregnant.

Certain pediatric iron supplements may be designed to fulfill the specific needs of children, particularly those who are at risk of iron deficiency.

Certain kinds of formulations of iron supplements may be necessary for those with medical problems like Crohn's disease or celiac disease that impact iron absorption. In these situations, speaking with a medical expert is crucial to choosing the right vitamin and dose.

Additionally, since non-heme iron from plants is not as easily absorbed as heme iron from animal products, vegetarians and vegans may need to pay particular attention to how much iron they consume. Iron-rich diets combined with sources of vitamin C can improve the absorption of non-heme iron. In certain situations, it could be advised for those who follow vegetarian or vegan diets to take iron supplements to make sure they are getting enough iron.

Contrasting Over-The-Counter And Prescription Iron Supplements

The decision between prescription and over-the-counter (OTC) iron supplements is based on the medical history and unique needs of the individual. Iron supplements are frequently accessible over-the-counter and without a prescription.

For people who are mildly iron deficient or as a preventative step, these over-the-counter vitamins are usually adequate.

They are usually convenient and well-tolerated.

A healthcare professional might suggest a prescription iron supplement, though, if the patient suffers from a more severe case of iron deficiency anemia or has underlying medical issues that interfere with iron metabolism or absorption.

Prescription iron supplements come in a variety of formats to meet specific needs and frequently have a greater elemental iron concentration.

selecting the appropriate iron supplement requires taking into account the kind of supplement, unique population requirements, and the choice between OTC and prescription solutions.

To choose the best iron supplement for your particular needs, you must speak with a healthcare provider.

They will consider your general health, your dietary choices, and the severity of your iron shortage. Sufficient consumption of iron is essential for general health and wellness, and iron deficiency anemia and associated disorders can be effectively treated with the appropriate supplement.

Relationships With Additional Nutrients

Interactions with other nutrients can also affect iron bioavailability and absorption:

Calcium: When taken in combination with non-heme iron, calcium can prevent both types of iron from being absorbed.

As a result, it's best to refrain from taking calcium-rich foods or supplements when eating meals high in iron.

Zinc: In the intestines, zinc and iron compete for absorption. Too much zinc can prevent the body from absorbing iron, therefore it's critical to consume both minerals in moderation.

Vitamin A: For the best iron absorption, a sufficient level of vitamin A is required. Iron utilization might be negatively impacted by a vitamin A deficit.

Folate: By promoting the synthesis of red blood cells, folate contributes to the metabolism of iron and may help avoid anemia. Sufficient consumption of folate can improve how well iron supplements work to treat iron-deficiency anemia.

maintaining appropriate iron levels in the body requires knowledge of the variables influencing iron absorption, application of techniques to increase iron bioavailability, and comprehension of the interactions between iron and other nutrients.

Ensuring optimal intake and utilization of iron can be achieved by a balanced diet, appropriate meal combinations, and attention to specific health concerns.

Iron Overload And Supplementation

A vital mineral, iron is necessary for several physiological functions, including the transport of oxygen, the synthesis of DNA, and the creation of energy.

However, because both an iron overload and a deficit can have detrimental effects on health, it is imperative to maintain the proper balance of iron in the body.

Iron supplements are frequently used to prevent iron deficiency anemia in those who are at risk or to treat iron deficiency anemia. On the other hand, using iron supplements excessively or carelessly might result in iron overload, a condition that carries several health hazards.

CHAPTER FIVE

Effects Of Iron Supplementation

Iron deficiency anemia, a disorder in which the body does not have enough iron to make enough red blood cells, is frequently treated with iron supplements. Although using iron supplements is generally safe and beneficial, there may be adverse effects. For those who are thinking about taking iron supplements or who are already taking them, knowing these side effects and how to handle them is crucial.

Typical Adverse Effects

Gastrointestinal Distress: This is one of the most typical adverse effects of taking iron supplements. This can involve symptoms like upset stomach, diarrhea, constipation, nausea, and abdominal discomfort. These symptoms could be brought on by the iron irritating the lining of the stomach and intestines or by the body having trouble absorbing it.

Dark feces: Iron supplements can make feces appear darker, usually taking on a green or black tint. The interaction between the unabsorbed iron and the natural hues in the stool causes this harmless side effect.

Taste Changes: When taking iron supplements, some people may notice an unpleasant or metallic taste in their mouth. Although this can be inconvenient, it is typically transient and manageable with the solutions we will cover later.

Rarely, people may develop allergic responses to iron supplements. These reactions might manifest as rash, itching, swelling, and breathing difficulties. It is necessary to seek emergency medical assistance if any of these symptoms appear.

Constipation: Some people may experience constipation as a result of taking iron supplements, which can make it difficult to have regular bowel movements. For people who are already prone to constipation, this can be very problematic.

Methods For Reducing Adverse Reactions

Split the Dose: Dividing the recommended daily intake of iron into two smaller doses helps reduce the risk of gastrointestinal adverse effects. The body may be able to absorb and tolerate the iron more easily as a result.

Consume with Food: Consuming iron supplements with food usually results in greater tolerance. Iron consumption with food can lessen the chance of an upset stomach.

Select the Correct Kind: Iron supplements come in a variety of forms, including ferrous fumarate, ferrous gluconate, and ferrous sulfate. It may be easier for some people to tolerate one type than another, so asking a healthcare professional for advice may be helpful.

Keep Yourself Hydrated: One common negative effect of iron supplements is constipation, which can be lessened by drinking lots of water. Bowel movements can be more comfortable and stools can be softened by drinking enough water.

Use Fiber: Increasing the amount of fiber in your diet helps both prevent and treat constipation. Foods and supplements high in fiber can encourage regular bowel motions.

Over-the-counter remedies: Certain iron supplement side effects may be managed with over-the-counter drugs like antacids or stool softeners, but only after consulting a healthcare professional.

When To Get Help From A Physician

Even while the majority of iron supplement side effects are moderate and controllable, there are several circumstances in which you should see a doctor right away. These consist of:

Severe Allergic Reactions: It's imperative to get emergency medical attention if you have symptoms such as breathing difficulties, facial or throat swelling, hives, or a severe rash.

Severe or Persistent Gastrointestinal Symptoms: You should get medical attention right away if you experience symptoms such as severe abdomen pain, blood in your stools, or persistent vomiting.

Iron Overdose: Immediate medical assistance is necessary in cases of accidental or deliberate iron overdose. Nausea, vomiting, diarrhea, lightheadedness, and in extreme situations, coma or even death, are possible symptoms.

Unexplained Symptoms: It's crucial to speak with a healthcare provider if you have unexplained symptoms while taking iron supplements. They can help you identify whether the symptoms are caused by iron supplementation or by an underlying medical problem.

While iron deficiency anemia can benefit from iron supplementation, there may be adverse effects. An individual can safely and successfully manage their iron supplements by being aware of these possible adverse effects and taking steps to reduce them. However, if you experience severe or uncommon symptoms due to iron supplementation, you should be cautious and seek medical assistance.

CHAPTER SIX

Iron And Medical Problems

One key mineral that is vital to sustaining healthy health is iron. It is a crucial part of several proteins and enzymes involved in vital metabolic activities, including hemoglobin, the protein in the blood that carries oxygen.

Nonetheless, there is a complicated relationship between iron and health, and the body may react negatively to both an excess or insufficient amount of iron.

Iron deficiency anemia is one of the most prevalent iron-related medical disorders. This happens when the body doesn't have enough iron to make enough hemoglobin, which causes symptoms including weakness, exhaustion, pale complexion, and decreased tolerance to exertion. Worldwide, iron deficiency anemia is common and can be brought on by several circumstances, such as poor iron absorption from food, insufficient dietary iron intake, or increased iron requirements as a result of pregnancy or a child's rapid growth.

Iron While Expecting

The body needs a lot more iron during pregnancy to sustain the developing fetus and the mother's increased blood volume. Both the developing child and the expectant mother require iron.

Because of these higher iron demands, pregnant women are more likely to develop iron deficiency anemia. Women are frequently advised to take iron supplements as a precaution against iron deficiency to guarantee a safe pregnancy.

Preterm birth and low birth weight are two consequences of anemia that can be avoided by taking iron supplements throughout pregnancy.

To make sure pregnant women are getting enough iron and to modify iron supplementation as needed, healthcare professionals must regularly check the iron levels of their patients.

However consuming too much iron when pregnant can result in iron overload, which can be dangerous. Finding the ideal balance is essential for the developing child's health as well as the mother's.

Children's Health And Iron

An essential component of a child's growth and development is iron. It is essential for the synthesis of hemoglobin, which carries oxygen to tissues and organs to maintain healthy function. Youngsters are especially susceptible to iron shortage because of their fast growth and frequently low-iron eating habits. Because they have little iron stores at birth and need a lot of iron for proper development, infants are especially vulnerable.

Insufficient iron intake in children can lead to delayed growth, reduced cognitive abilities, and heightened vulnerability to infections. Pediatric healthcare professionals frequently advise children who are at risk of iron deficiency—such as those who are prematurely born or have low birth weights—to take iron supplements and meals fortified with iron.

On the other hand, children should not consume too much iron since this might result in toxicity and other health problems.

Iron balance is important for general health and optimal performance for athletes and physically active people.

Because iron is essential for oxygen transport, muscles require more oxygen when exercise intensity rises.

Fatigue, poor endurance, and diminished exercise capacity might result from an iron shortage.

Due to increased iron losses through sweat and urine, athletes—especially those engaged in endurance sports like long-distance running or cycling—are more likely to develop iron insufficiency.

These people frequently have their iron levels checked regularly to identify iron deficiency early and implement corrective actions, such as changing their diets or taking supplements.

Iron is an essential mineral for good health in general, and the importance of iron increases when considering particular medical disorders.

To ensure that people may lead active, healthy lifestyles while fulfilling their specific iron needs, it is crucial to maintain an appropriate balance of iron during pregnancy, infancy, and in the context of athletic performance.

To properly traverse the complexities of iron and health, proper monitoring and advice from medical professionals are crucial.

Research And Future Paths

With continuous studies aiming at enhancing our knowledge of iron requirements, supplementation, and health effects, the field of iron supplementation is always changing.

To address the worldwide health burden of iron deficiency and anemia, these future research directions are essential.

CHAPTER SEVEN

Current Investigations Into Iron Supplementation

The main goals of ongoing research on iron supplementation are to improve present methods and address a range of issues related to iron intake and absorption.

One area of research studies the creation of alternative iron supplements, such as non-heme iron sources, that may be more bioavailable and have fewer side effects.

Researchers are also trying to decrease adverse effects and increase patient compliance by optimizing dose regimens.

Ongoing research examines the possible synergistic effects of mixing iron with other nutrients, such as vitamin C, which can improve iron absorption, in addition to iron supplement formulations. This method could result in better-supplementing plans, particularly for people with dietary restrictions or health issues that interfere with iron absorption.

Understanding the unique iron requirements for various population groups, taking into account variables like age, sex, and pregnancy, is another crucial component of research.

This work contributes to the customization of iron supplementation guidelines to better suit the demands of various demographics.

New Innovations And Trends

The future of iron supplementation is being shaped by several new developments and trends.

The investigation of iron supplies derived from plants is one noteworthy trend, particularly for vegans and vegetarians. Scholars are examining iron's bioavailability in plant-based diets and creating novel dietary approaches to improve iron absorption from these sources.

Other new trends include the utilization of genetic data and personalized diets. Researchers are looking into how a person's genetic composition may affect how much iron they require and how well they absorb it. This can result in suggestions for individualized iron supplementation that provides the appropriate amount and type of iron depending on a person's genetic profile.

Another cutting-edge field of iron supplementation study is nanotechnology. Researchers are working on producing iron particles at the nanoscale, which may have better bioavailability and fewer negative effects on the gastrointestinal tract. These developments have the potential to completely change the way iron supplements are taken, improving both their effectiveness and tolerability.

Prospective Future Advancements

Prospective advancements in iron supplementation in the future could lead to a variety of fascinating opportunities.

The creation of sophisticated iron delivery systems, such as liposomes, nanoparticles, or other encapsulation technologies, is one field of investigation.

These approaches have the potential to decrease side effects, increase supplemental convenience, and improve iron absorption.

Additionally, there is potential in the creation of iron-fortified meals that have better texture, taste, and nutritional absorption.

For small children and expectant mothers who might find it difficult to take conventional iron supplements, this could be helpful. Adding iron to frequently consumed foods may aid in addressing iron deficits in the general public.

The future of iron supplementation may also be greatly impacted by the incorporation of AI and machine learning into healthcare and nutrition. With the help of these technologies, those who are at risk of iron deficiency might be identified and therapies could be customized according to their dietary preferences and health information.

The future of iron supplementation is characterized by continued research aimed at improving current methods, discoveries in plant-based sources and tailored nutrition, and possible advancements in the form of AI-assisted interventions and sophisticated delivery systems.

These initiatives are critical to tackling the global public health issue of anemia and iron deficiency.

The exploration of these novel approaches holds promise for augmenting the efficiency and availability of iron supplementation, hence improving the health and welfare of people globally.

Choosing Knowledgeably

Maintaining excellent health requires making educated decisions about iron supplementation. An essential mineral, iron is necessary for many body processes, including the creation of red blood cells, the transportation of oxygen, and the synthesis of energy.

It's crucial to speak with medical professionals, determine your unique needs, and select the best type of iron supplement for you when thinking about taking one.

Collaborating With Medical Experts

It is strongly advised to speak with a healthcare provider, such as a doctor or qualified nutritionist, before beginning any iron supplementation program.

These professionals can evaluate your specific requirements, consider your medical background, and suggest the best course of action for iron supplementation. To assess your current iron levels and find any underlying medical issues that might be affecting your absorption of iron, they might also run blood tests on you.

You can ask medical specialists for advice on whether or not you need an iron supplement. Making dietary changes could sometimes be enough to meet your iron needs. If you require iron supplements, your doctor can advise you on the right kind and dose, making sure it is both safe and beneficial for your unique situation.

Striking The Correct Balance

When it comes to iron supplementation, several considerations need to be balanced. Determining the appropriate iron form, dosage, and supplementation period is critical. The amount needed can vary greatly based on the demands of the individual and the purpose of the supplement. For instance, different amounts may be needed for sportsmen, pregnant women, and those with iron-deficiency anemia.

Another important factor to think about is the type of iron supplement. Several types are accessible, including heme iron, ferrous gluconate, and ferrous sulfate.

Everyone has a different rate of absorption and possible adverse effects. Making the appropriate choice will maximize the positive consequences and reduce the negative ones.

The length of time that iron is supplemented also differs. While some people may need long-term or even lifetime supplementation, others may just need it temporarily to remedy an acute deficit. Maintaining the proper balance necessitates routine monitoring by medical experts who can modify the regimen as necessary.

Closing Reflections And Suggestions

Making wise choices and exercising prudence are important when it comes to iron supplements. The assistance of healthcare specialists is essential during this process. To find out if supplements are required and to get tailored advice, seek their expertise.

Take dosage, form, and duration into consideration while selecting an iron supplement.

Always heed the advice given to you by your healthcare practitioner and complete the recommended course of action. Maintain a well-balanced diet full of foods high in iron to support your supplementing.

Conclusion

To prevent iron-deficiency disorders and preserve optimal health, iron supplementation might be a useful strategy. Making wise decisions when it comes to iron supplements is crucial. Getting advice from medical experts, such as physicians or registered dietitians, is essential for figuring out what's best for you and your particular circumstances.

It is equally crucial to find the ideal balance for iron supplementation in terms of dosage, type, and duration.

You may make sure that your iron supplementation is safe, efficient, and customized to your unique situation by collaborating closely with your healthcare professional.

Your health and well-being are ultimately what matter most, and making wise decisions about iron supplements can help you reach and stay at your best.